HOW TO BURN BELLY FAT

EASY GUIDE ON WAYS TO BURN BELLY FAT

BLESSED VICTORY

COPYWRITE

INTRODUCTION

With the consumption of high-fat and trans-fat foods, many people have difficulty controlling the accumulation of fat around their abdomen, also known as belly fat. It is important to note that there are two types of belly fat, namely visceral and abdominal fat. Visceral fat, which surrounds a person's organs such as the liver, has been linked to several chronic diseases including metabolic syndrome, type 2 diabetes, heart disease, and certain types of cancer. On the other hand, abdominal fat is often more visible and can be improved through diet and exercise. Therefore, it is essential for people to focus on improving nutrition, increasing physical activity levels, and making other lifestyle changes in order to reduce their risk of developing chronic diseases due to excess belly fat.

CHAPTER ONE

Fat Around The Abdomen

Belly fat refers to fat around the abdomen. There are two types of belly fat:

Visceral: This fat surrounds a person's organs. Visceral refers to fat surrounding the liver and other abdominal organs. Having high levels of visceral fat is associated with an increased risk for chronic disease such as metabolic syndrome, type 2 diabetes, heart disease, and certain types of cancer.

Subcutaneous: This is fat that sits under the skin. Subcutaneous is the layer of fat that sits directly under the skin. This type is less harmful to health and serves as a layer of protection for your organs as well as insulation to regulate body temperature.

Having a high amount of subcutaneous fat is linked with a higher amount of visceral fat, therefore increasing your risk of health problems. Focusing on a health-promoting lifestyle, which helps prevent excessive amounts of both types of fat, is important.

Health complications from visceral fat are more harmful than having subcutaneous fat.

People can make many lifestyle and dietary changes to lose belly fat.

Why Is Belly Fat Dangerous?

Being overweight is one of the leading causes of major diseases.

Excess belly fat can increase the risk of:

- heart disease
- heart attacks
- high blood pressure
- stroke
- type 2 diabetes
- asthma
- breast cancer
- colon cancer
- dementia

CHAPTER TWO

Causes Of Belly Fat

Common causes of excess belly fat include:

1. Poor diet

Sugary food such as cakes and candy, and drinks such as soda and fruit juice, can:

- cause weight gain
- slow a person's metabolism
- reduce a person's ability to burn fat
- Low-protein, high-carb diets may also affect weight. Protein helps a person feel fuller for longer, and people who do not include lean protein in their diet may eat more food overall.
- Trans fats, in particular, can cause inflammation and may lead to obesity. Trans fats are in many foods, including fast food and baked goods like muffins and crackers.
- The American Heart Association Trusted Source recommends that people replace trans

fats with healthy whole-grain foods, monounsaturated fats, and polyunsaturated fats.

It is important to read food labels as they can help individuals better understand the ingredients and nutritional information in the food they consume. It is also important to be aware of how many added sugars one is consuming on a daily basis, as these can be found in many common foods such as baked goods, pastries, muffins, flavored yogurts, breakfast cereals, granola and protein bars, prepackaged foods, and sugar-sweetened beverages (SSBs). SSBs are particularly associated with an increase of visceral abdominal fat and should be limited as much as possible. Therefore, it is important to prioritize fresh and minimally processed foods over highly processed foods for a healthy diet.

SSBs are the largest contributor of sugar intake in the United States primarily due to their low cost, convenience, and ease of consumption. Unlike food, SSBs can be consumed quickly in large volumes since they require minimal processing.

Sugar sweetened beverages (SSB) are notorious for providing little to no nutritional value, despite the large intake of calories and sugar they offer. It is not uncommon for many individuals to consume multiple SSBs in a single day, for example two 16 fluid ounce (480 mL) bottles of soda can add up to 384 calories and 104 grams of sugar. This can pose a threat to one's health, especially when consumed alongside other processed foods with high sugar content, as it may lead to an excessive calorie intake and excess visceral fat. Furthermore, drinking your calories particularly from SSBs can lead to a temporary spike in blood sugar followed by a crash, leading to you feeling hungry quickly and needing to drink or eat soon again.

Though sugar-sweetened beverages (SSBs) have long been associated with visceral fat and weight gain, research suggests that regular sugar and high-fructose corn syrup both provide excessive calories to the body, leading to increases in weight. For this reason, it is best to limit SSBs to special occasions and opt for whole, minimally processed foods as well as water and unsweetened coffee/tea. Making these changes can help you maintain a healthier lifestyle and reduce your risk of gaining weight from sugar-sweetened beverages.

2. Too much alcohol

Consuming excess alcohol can cause a variety of health problems, including liver disease and inflammation.

Alcohol can have both healthful and harmful effects.

When consumed in moderate amounts, especially as red wine, it is associated with lower risk of heart disease.

However, high alcohol intake may lead to inflammation, liver disease, certain types of cancer, excess weight gain, and many other health problems.

Therefore, limiting alcohol consumption is an important strategy for controlling weight gain. The Centers for Disease Control and Prevention (CDC) recommend no more than one drink per day for women and two drinks per day for men, or avoiding alcohol completely. Alcohol contributes to weight gain due to its high calorie content (7 calories per gram) and many alcoholic beverages are high in sugar. Excessive alcohol consumption is associated with greater visceral fat accumulation and a higher body mass index (BMI). It's important to remember that even moderate amounts of alcohol can lead to weight gain, so limiting alcohol is key to maintaining a healthy weight.

Alcohol may increase appetite and decrease inhibitions, leading to greater overall calorie intake.

Not only can alcohol lead to poorer judgement and decreased fat oxidation, but it may also alter hormones related to hunger and fullness, which may lead to greater consumption of less nutritious foods. Moreover, there is evidence that alcohol consumption can increase cortisol levels, promoting abdominal fat storage. Furthermore, physical activity the day of and after drinking may be diminished due to consumption of alcohol, resulting in an increased risk for weight gain. Moreover, a recent review of 127 studies found a significant dose-dependent relationship between alcohol consumption and weight gain. Therefore, it is important to be aware of how alcohol consumption can contribute to weight gain.

Other studies have also shown a high alcohol intake (2–3 drinks or more per day) is linked to weight gain including abdominal obesity, especially in men.

If you choose to drink, aim for no more than 1–2 drinks per day.

A 2015 report on alcohol consumption and obesity found that drinking excess alcohol causes males to gain weight around their bellies, though study results in females are inconsistent.

3. Lack of exercise (Sedentary lifestyle and physical inactivity)

It is important to maintain a healthy lifestyle in order to prevent weight gain. An inactive lifestyle can lead to a sedentary one, as prolonged sitting throughout the day (e.g., watching TV, sitting at a work desk, long commutes, playing video games, etc.) can be detrimental to health. Even if a person is physically active, meaning they engage in physical labor or exercise, this may not be enough to prevent the risk of negative health events and weight gain. Therefore, it is important to ensure that you are engaging in physical activity regularly and managing your calorie intake in order to maintain a healthy lifestyle.

Additionally, research indicates that the majority of children and adults do not meet the recommended physical activity guidelines. In fact, up to 80% of adults do not meet the recommended aerobic and resistance training recommendations outlined in the Physical Activity Guidelines for Americans.

This indicates that Americans are becoming more and more sedentary, with a direct increase in abdominal fat due to a lack of physical activity. This poses a serious threat to the public health, as it is a major risk factor for many chronic diseases such as type 2 diabetes, coronary heart disease and stroke. To prevent these conditions, it's important to establish an active lifestyle and reduce inactivity levels, which can be done through regular exercise and movement throughout the day.

In one study, researchers reported that people who performed resistance or aerobic exercise for 1 year after losing weight were able to prevent regaining visceral fat, while those who did not exercise had a 25–38% increase in belly fat.

Another study showed that those who sat for over 8 hours each day (not including sleeping hours) had a 62% increased risk of obesity compared with those who sat for less than 4 hours each day.

It's recommended that most adults aim for at least 150 minutes of moderate aerobic physical activity (or 75 minutes of vigorous activity) each week and engage in regular resistance training.

Further, try to limit sedentary behaviors and prolonged sitting. If sitting is part of your work, try to incorporate "standing breaks" every 30–90 minutes by standing for 5–10 minutes or taking a quick walk around your office, home or neighborhood.

4. Stress and Cortisol

Cortisol is an important hormone for keeping us safe and healthy. In times of high stress or danger, it can help us cope and survive by releasing the necessary energy to help us through the situation. Unfortunately, this means that too much cortisol from a lifestyle of continuously being under pressure can be detrimental to our health. It can cause us to reach for food for comfort and store those excess calories around the belly, leading to weight gain. Therefore, it is essential to maintain a good balance in our lives by finding ways to reduce stress and manage our lifestyle better.

It's produced by the adrenal glands and is known as a "stress hormone" because it helps your body respond to a physical or psychological threat or stressor.

In this fast-paced society, it has become difficult to spend time in healthy, stress-reducing activities. The effects of chronic stress can be seen both mentally and physically, leading to an increased risk of negative health events and weight gain. Excess production of cortisol due to chronic stress can cause visceral fat to accumulate and make it harder to lose. Therefore, it is important to take steps towards a healthier lifestyle to reduce the impact of chronic stress on our bodies. Regular exercise, a balanced diet, and quality sleep are critical components in maintaining a healthy lifestyle. Furthermore, higher levels of cortisol in regard to food may lead some to choose high-calorie foods for comfort, which can lead to unwanted weight gain.

This can lead to overconsumption of foods high in fat and sugar, which are quick and dense forms of energy, to prepare the body for the perceived threat. Nowadays with chronic stress, this food is now used for comfort which can lead to overeating and eventually weight gain.

Additionally, chronic stress can affect other lifestyle behaviors that may lead to weight gain, such as negative coping behaviors (e.g., substance abuse), poor sleep quality, sedentary behaviors, and physical inactivity.

The relationship between stress and weight gain also seems to work in reverse, whereby having excess abdominal fat itself can increase cortisol levels, driving a negative cycle of chronic stress in the body.

Therefore, managing your stress through health-promoting lifestyle behaviors (e.g., nutrient-dense diet, regular exercise, meditation, addressing mental health) and working with a healthcare professional should be a priority.

5. Genetics

There is some evidence that a person's genes can play a part in whether they become obese. Scientists think genes can influence behavior, metabolism, and the risk of developing obesity-related diseases.

Genes play a major role in the risk of developing obesity.

Similarly, it appears that the tendency to store fat in the abdomen versus other parts of the body, is partly influenced by genetics.

Interestingly, recent research has started to identify single genes associated with obesity. For example, certain genes may influence the release and action of leptin, a hormone responsible for appetite regulation and weight management.

While promising, much more research needs to be conducted in this area.

Environmental factors and behavior also play a role in the likelihood of people becoming obese.

6. Poor sleep

A 2013 study Trusted Source links weight gain to short sleep duration, which could lead to an excess of belly fat. However, causality cannot be inferred from this study.

Short duration of sleep is linked to an increase in food intake, which may play a part in the development of abdominal fat.

Not getting enough good sleep also may, potentially, lead to unhealthy eating behaviors, such as emotional eating.

Getting enough sleep is crucial for your health.

Many studies have linked inadequate sleep with weight gain, which may include abdominal fat.

There are many potential causes of weight gain from lack of sleep, including increased food intake to compensate for lack of energy, changes in hunger hormones, inflammation, and lack of physical activity due to tiredness.

For example, those with inadequate sleep are more likely to select low-nutrient options (e.g., foods high in sugar and fat) and consume more calories daily than those who get enough sleep each night.

What's more, sleep disorders may also lead to weight gain. One of the most common disorders, sleep apnea, is a condition in which breathing stops repeatedly during the night due to soft tissue in the throat blocking the airway.

However, lack of sleep and weight gain present a "chicken or the egg" scenario. While sleep deprivation appears to contribute to weight gain, higher BMIs can lead to sleep issues and sleep disorders

7. Smoking

Researchers may not consider smoking to be a direct cause of belly fat, but they do believe it to be a risk factor.

A 2012 study published in the journal PloS one Trusted Source showed that, although obesity was the same between smokers and nonsmokers, smokers had more belly and visceral fat than nonsmokers.

8. Trans fats

Trans fats are the among the unhealthiest fats.

While small amounts of trans fat occur in nature, they're mainly created for the food system by adding hydrogen to unsaturated fats in order to make them more stable and allow them to be solid at room temperature.

Trans fats are often used in baked products and packaged foods as a cheap yet effective replacement for butter, lard, and higher-cost items.

Artificial trans fats have been shown to cause inflammation, which can lead to insulin resistance, heart disease, certain types of cancer, and various other diseases. However, ruminant trans fats, which are found naturally in dairy and meat products, do not have the same negative health effects.

The American Heart Association recommends severely limiting or completely avoiding artificial trans fats. Many countries, including the United States and Canada, have banned the use of trans fats in food products due to their adverse effects on health.

Though it's thought that trans fat may also contribute to visceral fat and has been attributed to poor health over recent decades there's little recent research on the topic.

Even with many countries having taken steps to limit or ban the use of artificial trans fats in the food supply, it's important to still check the nutrition label if you're unsure.

9. Menopause

Gaining belly fat during menopause is extremely common.

At puberty, the hormone estrogen signals the body to begin storing fat on the hips and thighs in preparation for a potential pregnancy. This subcutaneous fat isn't harmful from a health standpoint, although it can be difficult to lose in some cases

Menopause officially occurs one year after a woman has her last menstrual period. Around this time, estrogen levels drop dramatically. Though menopause affects all women differently, in general it tends to cause fat to be stored in the abdomen, rather than on the hips and thighs.

While menopause is a completely natural part of the aging process, interventions such as estrogen therapy may lower your risk of abdominal fat storage and its associated health risks.

If you have concerns, speak with a healthcare professional or a registered dietitian nutritionist.

10. The wrong gut bacteria

Hundreds of types of bacteria live in your gut, mainly in your colon. Some of these bacteria benefit health, while others can cause problems.

Gut bacteria are collectively known as your gut flora or microbiome. Gut health is important for maintaining a healthy immune system and decreasing disease risk.

While the connection between the gut microbiome and health continues to be investigated, current research suggests imbalances in gut bacteria may increase your risk of developing a number of diseases, including type 2 diabetes, heart disease, obesity, and gut disorders (e.g., irritable bowel syndrome, inflammatory bowel disease)

There's also some research suggesting that having an unhealthy balance of gut bacteria may promote weight gain, including abdominal fat. In particular, having a higher ratio of Firmicutes bacteria to Bacteroidetes is associated with higher weight and visceral fat.

It's thought that changes in bacteria diversity may lead to changes in energy and nutrient metabolism, stimulate inflammation, and alter hormone regulation, leading to weight gain. That said, further research into this topic is needed.

One randomized, double-blind 12-week study in postmenopausal women with obesity showed that taking a probiotic containing five strains of "good" bacteria led to significant reductions in body fat percentage and visceral fat. However, the small group size and uncontrolled diet posed limitations.

Further, a 2018 review of studies involving 957 people showed probiotic supplementation was significantly associated with lower BMI, body fat percentage, and visceral fat. The effect sizes were small, meaning the results may not be clinically meaningful.

While there appears to be a relationship between gut microbiome diversity and visceral fat, more research is needed to best understand its relationship and which interventions and probiotic strains may be most effective.

Additionally, in general, eating a low fiber diet high in sugar and saturated fat tends to be linked to unhealthy gut bacteria, whereas a fiber-dense diet rich in fruits and vegetables and whole, minimally processed foods seems to create a healthy gut.

11. Low fiber diet

Fiber is incredibly important for optimal health and weight management.

Some types of fiber can help you feel full, stabilize hunger hormones, and manage hunger (86).

In an observational study involving 1,114 men and women, soluble fiber intake was associated with reduced abdominal fat. For each 10-gram increase in soluble fiber, there was a 3.7% decrease in belly fat accumulation.

Diets high in refined carbs and low in fiber appear to have the opposite effect on appetite and weight gain, including increases in belly fat.

One large study involving 2,854 adults found that high-fiber whole grains were associated with reduced abdominal fat, while refined grains were linked to increased abdominal fat.

Foods high in fiber include:

- beans
- lentils
- whole grains
- oats
- vegetables
- fruit
- plain popcorn
- nuts

• seeds

CHAPTER THREE

How to lose belly fat

The following steps may help people lose unwanted belly fat:

1. Improving their diet

A healthy, balanced diet can help a person lose weight, and is also likely to have a positive effect on their overall health.

People may want to avoid sugar, fatty foods, and refined carbohydrates that have low nutritional content. Instead, they can eat plenty of fruit and vegetables, lean proteins, and complex carbohydrates.

2. Reducing alcohol consumption

A person trying to lose excess abdominal fat can monitor their alcohol intake. Alcoholic drinks often contain additional sugar, which can contribute to weight gain.

3. Increasing exercise

A sedentary lifestyle can lead to many serious health problems, including weight gain. People trying to lose weight should include a good amount of exercise in their daily routine.

Undertaking both aerobic exercise and strength training can help people tackle their belly fat.

4. Getting more sunlight

A 2016 review indicates that exposure to sunlight in animals could lead to a reduction in weight gain and metabolic dysfunction.

The review notes that few studies have looked at the effects of sunlight on humans with respect to weight gain, and that more research is required.

5. Meditation

Stress can cause a person to gain weight. The release of the stress hormone cortisol influences a person's appetite and could cause them to eat more.

Stress-relieving tactics include mindfulness and meditation, and gentle exercise like yoga.

6. Improving sleep patterns

Sleep is vital to people's overall health.

Sleep's primary purpose is to allow the body to rest, heal, and recover, but it can also affect a person's weight.

Getting enough quality sleep is essential when a person is trying to shed weight, including belly fat.

7. Quitting smoking

Smoking is a risk factor for increased belly fat, as well as many other serious health concerns. Quitting can significantly reduce the risk from excess belly fat, as well as improve overall health.

CHAPTER FOUR

The Pros and Cons of Gummies for Weight Loss in Older Women

Gummies are a popular weight-loss supplement, and it's easy to see why. They are simple to use and do not necessitate any special equipment or exercise. Despite their popularity, there are some important factors to consider when using gummies for weight loss.

Weight loss gummies claim to help you lose weight in a variety of ways. Some gummies claim to suppress hunger, while others claim to increase metabolism. Some gummies also contain fat-burning ingredients such as green tea extract, garcinia cambogia, or hoodia gordonii. Despite these claims, there is little scientific evidence to back up the effectiveness of weight loss.

pros: One of the primary benefits of gummies is their ease of use. They are small and portable, making them ideal for on-the-go use. They are also simple to incorporate into one's daily routine because they are simply taken like any other supplement. Gummies also have the potential to provide health benefits. Gummies may help people lose weight more easily by suppressing appetite or increasing metabolism.

Cons: Despite the potential advantages, there are some disadvantages to using gummies for weight loss. There is no guarantee that gummies will actually help people lose weight because there is no scientific evidence to support their effectiveness. Another disadvantage is the possibility of side effects, as some gummies may contain ingredients that can interact with other medications or cause adverse reactions in some people. Furthermore, gummies can be quite costly, making them a less cost-effective option for weight loss than exercise.

Gummies vs. Exercise for Obese Older Women

Older women have two options for losing weight: gummies or exercise. Both options have advantages and disadvantages that must be considered in order to determine which option is best for each individual.

Gummies are convenient because they can be taken anywhere and do not require any physical effort. However, there is a lack of scientific evidence to back up their claims, and they may have unintended consequences. Exercise, on the other hand, provides numerous advantages, including improved overall health, increased muscle mass, and long-term weight loss. However, exercise has its own set of difficulties, such as the risk of injury, the difficulty in finding time, and the cost.

The best weight loss option will be determined by each individual's unique situation. Gummies may be a good option for older women looking for convenience and ease of use. Exercise, on the other hand, is a better option for older women looking for a more effective way to lose weight and improve their overall health. Ultimately, the ideal alternative will be determined by each individual's needs, preferences, and physical capabilities.

Regardless of which choice they pick, it is critical for older women to discover a weight loss method that works for them. This may entail experimenting with different tactics, such as mixing gummies with exercise or modifying their workout program to better suit their needs. The aim is to discover a solution that is long-term and allows people to lose weight while improving their overall health. Finally, the most essential thing is to discover a method that works for each individual and helps them to attain their weight loss objectives in a safe and lasting manner.

Feature	Gummies	Exercise
Convenience	High	Low
Ease of Use	High	Low
Scientific Evidence	Low	High
Cost	Varies, but can be expensive	Varies, but can be expensive
Potential Side Effects	Yes	No
Potential Benefits	Improved digestion, appetite control	Improved overall health, increased muscle mass, sustained weight loss
Potential Drawbacks	Lack of scientific evidence, potential side effects, and cost	Risk of injury, difficulty in finding time, and cost

When it comes to choosing between gummies and exercise for weight loss in older women, it is important to consider the benefits and drawbacks of each option. While gummies are convenient and easy to use, they may not be backed by scientific evidence and can be expensive. On the other hand, exercise offers a range of health benefits, but it can be challenging to start and maintain an exercise routine, especially for older women. Ultimately, the best approach for fat older women will depend on their individual needs, preferences, and health condition.

In conclusion, it is important to consider all options when looking for a solution to weight loss in older women. While gummies may be a convenient option, exercise is a more effective and sustainable way to improve overall health and achieve weight loss goals. Fat older women should speak to their doctor before starting any weight loss program, and get guidance on the best approach for their individual needs and health conditions.

CHAPTER FIVE

Is There Really 'One Trick' To Losing Belly Fat?

If an ad claims a "one-trick" solution, remember that its main purpose is to sell a product, not to help you. Because it's hard, good marketing means messaging. That's why they focus on trends, which piques your curiosity and leads you to click on the link and go to their site.

So, no, there`s not. But here's what you can do.

1. just start

There are usually a lot of things you need to improve to lose belly fat.But first, focus on changing or improving just one thing. After completing the first goal, you can move on to the next.

2. Target sugar

A good starting point for improving your dietary choices is to give up sugary drinks. Not just carbonated drinks, but juices as well. Sugar increases belly fat and fiber reduces belly fat. Therefore, juicing the fruit removes the fiber and leaves the pure sugars. So a very specific quick fix is   to give up sugary drinks.

Replacing sugary drinks with water can significantly reduce your sugar intake. Take that step and you'll know how to cut down on sugary foods.

If you have a sweet tooth and want to add to your meal, try apples, melons, or fresh berries. Remember that fruits do not replace vegetables.

3. Go Mediterranean

The popular "flat belly diet" incorporates much of the wisdom found in the Mediterranean diet to support everything from brain health to heart health. A basic requirement for both diets is to eat foods high in monosaturated fats (MUFAs), which help reduce abdominal fat accumulation.

MUFA-rich foods include olive oil, nuts and seeds, and avocados. , fish, etc. Regular consumption of yogurt has also been shown to help reduce belly fat.

Another nutrition trend that promises success when it comes to belly fat:

The Apple Cider Vinegar Diet. Animal studies have shown promise, but current human studies have yet to show impressive results.However, the data supporting the benefits of the Mediterranean diet are real. and is the reason for some dietary changes.

4. Front-load your meals

Whether it's a vegetable soup or an appetizer plate of vegetables, start your meal, especially the largest meal, with seasoned vegetables. And remember that vegetables should always occupy at least half of your plate and should be a mixture of starchy (like potatoes) and non-starchy (leafy greens, broccoli, etc.).

Eating vegetables first leaves less room for other unhealthy foods because they are full of plant fiber.

5. Commit to a physical lifestyle

The most important thing people can do to prevent belly fat buildup and get rid of existing belly fat is physical activity and even a better physical lifestyle. Visceral fat is the first fat to be lost during exercise for both men and women.

In some ways, moderate-intensity physical activity is the "magic pill" that many people seek. Because the health benefits don't stop at slimming your waistline.

In addition to reducing the risk of cancer, stroke, diabetes, and heart attack, research has shown that physical activity can significantly improve mood in people with major depressive disorder.

However, overtraining can lead to overproduction of cholesterol, which can be problematic when it comes to fighting belly fat.Excess levels of this stress hormone have been linked to belly fat.

Simply walking briskly an hour each day can have an impact by boosting your metabolism, as can adding an incline to your treadmill routine.

The bottom line is that when it comes to belly fat, the answer is not in drugs or supplements.

6. Move around, fidget

Here's something else most people probably don't know: Fidgeting is good for you. It's considered a non-exercise physical activity, and it's an important way to burn energy. You get more health benefits if, in addition to exercising, you are a more fidgety, more active person the rest of the day. This means gesturing while you're talking, tapping your foot, just moving around.

7. And try not to sit too much

Studies have shown that people who sit eight to nine hours a day, even if they exercise the recommended 150 minutes per week, do not get the same benefits of exercising as people who are more active throughout the day.

If you have to sit most of the day for your job, try to find some ways to move:

• Take small breaks throughout the day to walk around

• Use your lunch hour to take a longer walk

• Take the stairs instead of the elevator, if possible

• Do stretching exercises at your desk

• Just do your best to move around as much as you can

8. Redefine 'rest'

Having an active hobby and if you don't already have one, developing one is important. Get engaged in some kind of sport, whether it's a group activity or something you can do alone. Essentially, if an activity is pleasant to you, you'll continue to do it.

If your leisure time involves sitting around on the sofa or in a chair, you might actually be offsetting the positive health effects of exercising even if you're working out regularly.

Unfortunately, the general understanding of rest is relaxing in front of TV or dining out what we call "passive rest." But really, our rest should consist of sleep, and our leisure time should consist of fun physical activity, which is active rest.

Statistics suggest that out of 900 months in his life, the average man in the U.S. spends approximately 198 months watching TV, five months complaining about his boss, and five months waiting on hold.

Think of the other things you could do with those 208 months of your life. You could find activities that are better for your health and will help keep the belly fat away.

9. Don't rely on sit-ups to give you a six-pack

Unfortunately, sit-ups and crunches can't eliminate visceral fat directly. You can't reduce fat from specific parts of your body by exercising that body part; our bodies simply don't work that way.

With sit-ups or other abdominal exercises, you're toning the abdominal muscles but not burning intra-abdominal fat. The key is to lower your overall body fat with moderate-intensity physical activity and a healthy diet; when you reduce your total body fat, you'll also be reducing your belly fat.

So if you want to do abdominal exercises, make them part of your fitness routine. Just don't treat them as a substitute for the recommended 150 minutes of weekly moderate-intensity physical activity.

10. Develop more muscle

While sit-ups can't "target" belly fat, what they can do is help you burn calories, strengthen your core and develop more muscle. Because muscle is more metabolically active than fat, the more muscle you have, the more calories you'll burn when you're at rest.

You can also try lifting heavier weights and resting less between repetitions, which can promote calorie burning after you leave the gym.

Burning those extra calories can help you achieve and maintain a healthier weight in conjunction with regular cardiovascular exercise and a healthy diet.

11. Get some sleep

A recent study of 70,000 individuals showed that those getting less than five hours of sleep were more likely to gain 30 or more pounds.

12. Forget about weight loss drugs or supplements claiming 'one trick'

So far, there is not one single drug that is approved by the Federal Drug Administration for the reduction of belly fat. Supplements claiming a "one trick solution" to belly fat are not strictly regulated, and a lot of the claims made in the ads are not backed up by research.

The bottom line is that when it comes to belly fat, the answer is not in drugs or supplements. Enjoying a healthy lifestyle should be the focus. And while that's not as simple as swallowing a pill, the benefits will last a lifetime.

www.ingramcontent.com/pod-product-compliance
Lightning Source LLC
Chambersburg PA
CBHW061601250726
48657CB00020B/1006